Understanding the Autophagy Process in Humans

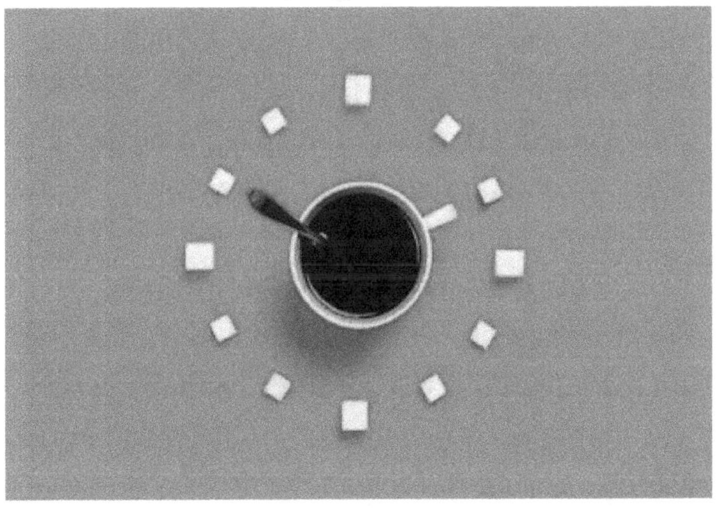

17-Hour Water Fasting Book Guide for Weight Loss, Anti-Aging, Detoxing, and Inner Cells Healing

Monica Meskill

Copyright © [2024], Monica Meskill,
All rights reserved.

<u>This book is a work of nonfiction</u>.

The information contained in this book is based on the author's personal experiences, research, and opinions. While the author has made every effort to ensure the accuracy of the information in this book, the author and publisher assume no responsibility for errors, omissions, or any damages resulting from the use of the information contained herein.

Table of contents

Understanding the Autophagy Process in Humans

17-Hour Water Fasting Book Guide for Weight Loss, Anti-Aging, Detoxing, and Inner Cells Healing

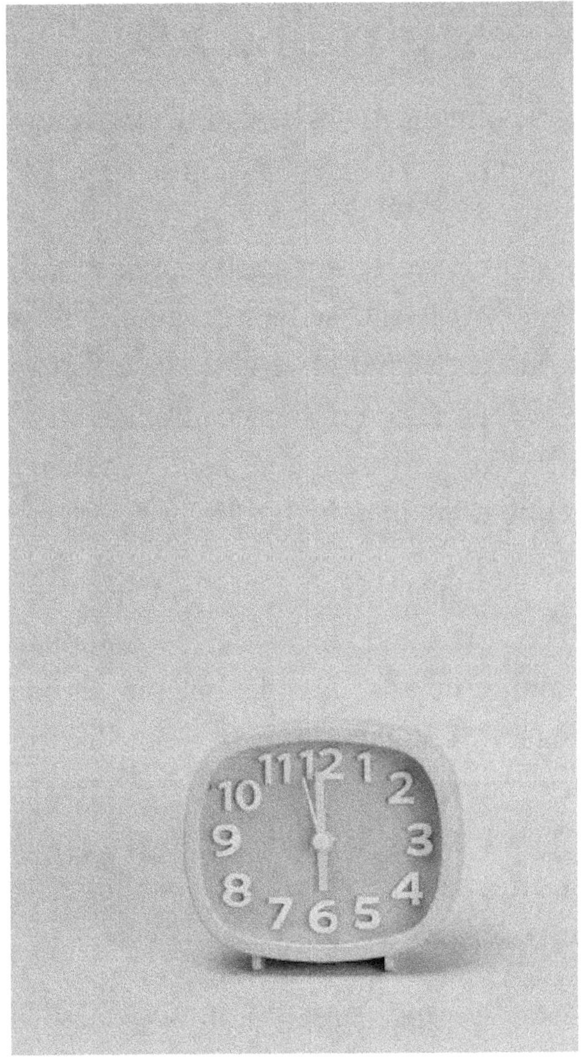

Introduction

In a bustling city where life moved at an unrelenting pace, lived Zarina, a woman grappling with the consequences of her dietary choices. For years, her daily routine had been entangled with the seductive allure of sugary treats and convenience foods. The effects of her lifestyle manifested in her health, and she found herself constantly fatigued, lacking vitality, and struggling to maintain a healthy weight.

Zarina had heard about the importance of a balanced diet and the role of autophagy in maintaining cellular health, but the temptations of sugary delights proved too formidable. Despite numerous attempts to curb her sweet tooth and adopt a healthier lifestyle, she found herself trapped in a cycle of indulgence and guilt.

One day, as she browsed through the virtual aisles of an online bookstore, she stumbled upon a book that promised a transformative journey: *"Understanding the Autophagy in Humans: A*

17-Hour Water Fasting Book Guide for Weight Loss, Anti-Aging, Detoxing, and Inner Cells Healing" by Monica Meskill. Intrigued by the title and desperate for change, Zarina decided to give it a chance.

As she delved into the pages of Monica Meskill's book, a revelation unfolded. The book not only explained the science behind autophagy in a clear and accessible manner but also provided practical guidance on implementing a 17-hour water fasting routine. Zarina learned about the impact of excessive sugar intake on the autophagy process and how adopting healthier dietary habits could unleash the body's innate healing mechanisms.

Motivated by newfound knowledge and armed with practical strategies from the book, Zarina embarked on a transformative journey. The 17-hour water fasting regimen became a cornerstone of her lifestyle, replacing the habitual sugar-laden snacks with nourishing alternatives. Slowly but steadily, Zarina noticed positive changes in her energy levels, weight, and overall well-being.

The book became her trusted companion, guiding her through the challenges of breaking old habits and embracing a healthier way of life. Zarina's story became a testament to the transformative power of understanding autophagy and making informed choices about diet and lifestyle.

Over time, Zarina not only regained control over her diet but also experienced the profound benefits of autophagy—weight loss, enhanced energy, and a radiant sense of vitality. Her journey, inspired by the wisdom imparted by Monica Meskill's book, became a beacon of hope for others seeking a path to better health through understanding and harnessing the body's natural processes.

The History behind Autophagy

Autophagy, a term derived from the Greek words **"auto,"** meaning **"self,"** and **"phagy,"** meaning **"eating,"** is a fundamental cellular process that plays a pivotal role in maintaining the health and functionality of our cells. It is a finely orchestrated mechanism through which cells remove damaged or dysfunctional components, allowing for recycling and renewal. This process is not only essential for cellular maintenance but also holds profound implications for overall human health.

In the journey of understanding autophagy, it is crucial to delve into the intricate machinery that governs this process. At its core, autophagy involves the engulfment and degradation of cellular components, such as organelles or proteins, within specialized structures known as autophagosomes. These cellular "cleanup crews" are deployed in response to various cues, including nutrient deprivation, stress, or cellular damage.

As we unravel the mysteries of autophagy, we discover its multifaceted benefits to the human body. Beyond mere cellular housekeeping, autophagy has been linked to a myriad of health benefits, ranging from weight management to anti-aging and even the facilitation of cellular detoxification. Understanding the molecular intricacies of autophagy allows us to appreciate its role in promoting longevity, resilience, and overall well-being.

This introduction sets the stage for an exploration of the science behind autophagy, its mechanisms, and its potential applications for human health. As we embark on this journey, we aim to demystify autophagy. We provide readers with a comprehensive guide to harnessing its power through practices like *17-hour water fasting for weight loss, anti-aging, detoxing, and inner cell healing*.

Importance of Understanding Autophagy in Humans

Understanding autophagy in humans is of paramount importance due to its central role in maintaining cellular health, influencing overall well-being, and potentially impacting the prevention of various diseases.

Here are key points highlighting the significance of comprehending autophagy:

→ **Cellular Maintenance and Renewal**: Autophagy serves as a crucial mechanism for removing damaged organelles, proteins, and other cellular components. This process ensures that cells remain functional and free from accumulated debris, contributing to cellular longevity and optimal performance.

→ **Adaptation to Stress and Nutrient Deprivation**: Autophagy plays a vital role in helping cells adapt to periods of stress in helping cells adapt to periods of stress or nutrient scarcity. During fasting or other challenging conditions, the recycling of cellular material through autophagy provides a source of energy and essential building blocks, enabling cells to endure and recover.

→ **Immune System Support**: Autophagy is implicated in the regulation of the immune system. It helps eliminate intracellular pathogens and supports the proper functioning of immune cells. Understanding autophagy is essential for comprehending how the body defends itself against infections and maintains immune homeostasis.

→ **Prevention of Neurodegenerative Diseases**: Research suggests a connection between impaired autophagy and the development of neurodegenerative disorders, such as Alzheimer's and Parkinson's disease. Understanding autophagy provides insights into potential therapeutic strategies for preventing or mitigating these conditions.

→ **Cancer Prevention**: Proper autophagic function is associated with the suppression of tumor development. Understanding how autophagy influences the regulation of cell growth and the removal of damaged cells helps in exploring avenues for cancer prevention and treatment.

→ **Metabolic Health and Weight Regulation**: Autophagy plays a role in regulating metabolic processes, including glucose and lipid metabolism. Understanding autophagy is crucial for comprehending how it affects body weight, insulin sensitivity, and overall metabolic health.

→ **Anti-Aging Benefits**: Autophagy has been linked to processes that may contribute to slowing down the aging of cells. By understanding and promoting autophagy, individuals may potentially support anti-aging mechanisms, leading to enhanced longevity and vitality.

In conclusion, understanding autophagy in humans is not only a key aspect of cellular biology but also holds immense implications for health and disease. From cellular maintenance to immune function and disease prevention, the knowledge of autophagy opens avenues for developing strategies to optimize health and potentially extend the quality of life.

Purpose and Scope of the Book

The main purpose and scope of the book titled "*Understanding the Autophagy in Humans: 17-Hour Water Fasting Book Guide for Weight Loss, Anti-Aging, Detoxing, and Inner Cells Healing*" are to provide readers with a comprehensive and accessible guide to the science of autophagy and its practical applications for improving various aspects of human health.

The book aims to achieve the following:

→ **Educate on Autophagy**: Provide a clear and understandable explanation of the concept of autophagy, detailing the molecular mechanisms and processes involved in cellular self-cleansing and renewal.

→ **Highlight Health Benefits**: Explore and emphasize the diverse health benefits associated with autophagy, including weight loss, anti-aging effects, detoxification, and inner cell healing.

The book aims to connect the understanding of autophagy with tangible outcomes that readers can achieve.

→ **Introduce 17-Hour Water Fasting**: Specifically, focus on the practice of 17-hour water fasting as a method to trigger and enhance autophagy. The book aims to guide readers through the principles and practicalities of incorporating this fasting regimen into their lifestyles.

→ **Provide Practical Guidance**: Offer practical tips, strategies, and guidance for individuals looking to implement 17-hour water fasting effectively. This includes information on how to overcome challenges, maintain nutritional balance, and adopt a sustainable approach to fasting.

→ **Address Specific Health Concerns**: Tailor information to address common health concerns related to diet, sugar intake, and overall well-being. The book aims to serve as a resource for individuals seeking solutions to specific health issues through the lens of autophagy.

→ **Empower Readers to Make Informed Choices**: Empower readers with knowledge that enables them to make informed choices about their dietary habits and lifestyle. By understanding the science of autophagy, readers can take proactive steps toward optimizing their health and well-being.

→ **Encourage Holistic Health Practices**: Advocate for a holistic approach to health, emphasizing the interconnectedness of diet, fasting, and cellular processes. The book aims to inspire readers to adopt a lifestyle that supports not only physical health but also longevity and vitality.

In summary, the purpose and scope of the book revolve around demystifying autophagy, connecting it to practical health outcomes, and guiding readers through the implementation of a 17-hour water-fasting approach. The overarching goal is to empower individuals to take control of their health by leveraging the principles of autophagy for a more vibrant and resilient life.

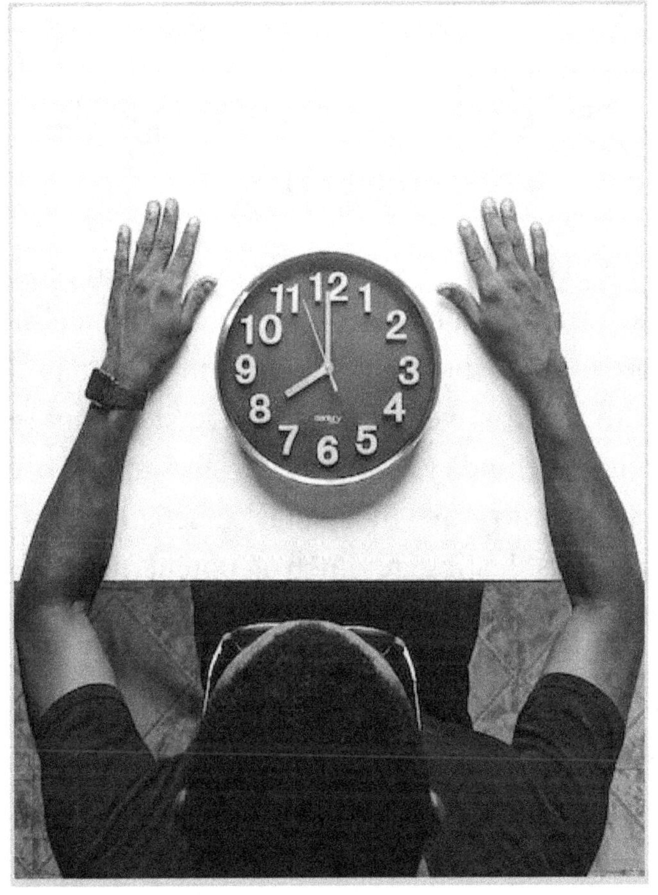

Chapter 1: The Science Behind 17-Hour Water Fasting

The practice of 17-hour water fasting is rooted in the intricate science of autophagy, a cellular process that holds profound implications for health and well-being. Understanding the science behind 17-hour water fasting involves delving into the molecular mechanisms that make this fasting regimen a potent trigger for autophagy.

Here's an exploration of the key scientific aspects:

→ **Nutrient Sensing and Autophagy Activation**: When the body enters a fasting state, especially during extended periods such as a 17-hour water fast, nutrient-sensing pathways are influenced. Specifically, the reduction in nutrient availability, particularly glucose and amino acids, activates pathways such as mTOR (mammalian target of rapamycin) inhibition. This serves as a crucial signal for the initiation of autophagy.

→ **AMP-Activated Protein Kinase (AMPK) Activation**: Fasting induces the activation of AMPK, a cellular energy sensor. AMPK activation is associated with increased autophagy, as it signifies a shift in cellular metabolism towards energy conservation and recycling. This activation is integral to the autophagic response during fasting.

→ **Energy Deprivation and Autophagic Flux**: The absence of external nutrient sources during a 17-hour water fast leads to a state of energy deprivation within cells. In response, cells initiate autophagic flux, a dynamic process involving the formation of autophagosomes, cargo recognition, and fusion with lysosomes. This flux facilitates the breakdown of cellular components for energy production.

→ **Enhanced Mitochondrial Autophagy (Mitophagy):** Fasting has been shown to stimulate mitophagy, a specialized form of autophagy targeting damaged or dysfunctional mitochondria. This process is crucial for maintaining cellular energy balance and preventing the accumulation of compromised cellular components.

→ **Regulation of Insulin and Insulin-Like Growth Factor-1 (IGF-1):** Fasting, particularly intermittent fasting, has been linked to improved insulin sensitivity and reduced levels of IGF-1. These hormonal changes contribute to autophagy induction, as insulin and IGF-1 signaling are known to inhibit autophagy.

→ **Protein Deacetylation and Sirtuin Activation:** Fasting promotes protein deacetylation, mediated by sirtuins, a class of enzymes with roles in cellular regulation. Sirtuin activation is associated with increased autophagy, further contributing to the cellular cleansing process.

→ **DNA Repair and Cellular Resilience**: Autophagy is involved in DNA repair processes, aiding in the maintenance of genomic stability. Fasting-induced autophagy enhances cellular resilience by addressing DNA damage and promoting the survival of healthy cells.

Understanding the science behind 17-hour water fasting reveals a sophisticated interplay of cellular signaling pathways, energy-sensing mechanisms, and orchestrated responses that collectively contribute to the activation of autophagy. This process, triggered by extended fasting, represents a powerful tool for cellular rejuvenation, detoxification, and the promotion of overall health and longevity.

Exploring Autophagy and Cellular Renewal

Autophagy, in its essence, unfolds as a captivating process within cells, intricately tied to the concept of cellular renewal. The beauty lies in the orchestrated dance of cellular components, where old and damaged structures are gracefully removed, making way for rejuvenation and optimal functioning.

Let's delve into the beauty of exploring autophagy and its profound connection to cellular renewal:

→ **Cellular Housekeeping**: Autophagy acts as the diligent custodian of the cell, engaging in a meticulous cleanup of cellular clutter. It selectively targets worn-out organelles, misfolded proteins, and other cellular debris for removal, leaving behind a refreshed and rejuvenated cellular environment.

→ **Balancing Act of Degradation and Recycling**: The beauty of autophagy lies in its ability to delicately balance the degradation of cellular components with the recycling of their building blocks. This recycling process ensures that valuable resources are not wasted, contributing to the sustainable upkeep of the cell.

→ **Adaptation to Changing Cellular Needs**: Autophagy is not a static process; it dynamically adapts to the changing needs of the cell. Whether responding to nutrient scarcity, stress, or other environmental cues, autophagy ensures that the cellular machinery remains flexible and resilient.

→ **Mitochondrial Quality Control through Mitophagy**: The beauty of autophagy extends to specialized forms such as mitophagy, which focuses on the selective removal of damaged mitochondria. This targeted quality control mechanism is crucial for maintaining energy balance and preventing the buildup of dysfunctional cellular powerhouses.

→ **Cleansing for Cellular Longevity**: Autophagy emerges as a fountain of youth for cells, contributing to their longevity and sustained functionality. By ridding cells of accumulated damage over time, autophagy plays a key role in supporting cellular health and potentially extending the lifespan of cells.

→ **Supporting Cellular Resilience**: Autophagy is not merely a process of removal; it actively participates in building cellular resilience. By repairing damaged cellular components and contributing to DNA repair processes, autophagy fortifies cells against the ravages of time and environmental stressors.

→ **A Symphony of Molecular Players**: Within the intricacies of autophagy, a symphony of molecular players orchestrates this ballet of renewal. From autophagosomes forming around cellular cargo to the fusion with lysosomes where degradation occurs, each step is a harmonious collaboration ensuring the cell's vitality.

→ **Harmony between Autophagy and Cellular Functions**: The beauty lies in the seamless integration of autophagy with various cellular functions. It doesn't disrupt cellular harmony but, instead, enhances it. Autophagy ensures that the balance between growth, maintenance, and renewal is finely tuned, contributing to overall cellular homeostasis.

In essence, exploring autophagy and cellular renewal unveils the marvels of nature's design at the microscopic level. It's a narrative of cellular resilience, adaptability, and perpetual renewal, echoing the beauty inherent in the sustained vitality of life at its most fundamental level.

Benefits of 17-Hour Fasting for Weight Loss

1. **Enhanced Fat Burning**: During a 17-hour fast, the body depletes its glycogen stores, prompting a shift to fat as the primary energy source. This promotes fat burning, aiding in weight loss by utilizing stored fat for energy.

2. **Caloric Restriction without Deprivation**: The restricted eating window in a 17-hour fast naturally limits calorie intake. This caloric restriction contributes to weight loss without the need for strict dieting, offering a sustainable approach.

3. **Improved Insulin Sensitivity**: Fasting periods enhance insulin sensitivity, meaning the body utilizes insulin more effectively to manage blood sugar. Improved insulin sensitivity is associated

with better weight management and reduced fat storage.

4. **<u>Increased Metabolic Rate</u>**: Short-term fasting has been linked to an increase in metabolic rate. This boost in metabolism can contribute to more efficient calorie burning, supporting weight loss efforts.

5. **<u>Activation of Autophagy</u>**: Fasting triggers autophagy, the cellular cleaning process that removes damaged cellular components. This not only supports overall health but may also indirectly contribute to weight loss by optimizing cellular function.

6. **<u>Reduction in Appetite Hormones</u>**: Fasting has been shown to impact hormones related to appetite regulation, such as ghrelin. Lower levels of appetite-stimulating hormones may lead to reduced overall calorie intake, aiding in weight loss.

7. **<u>Stabilization of Blood Sugar Levels</u>**: Fasting helps regulate blood sugar levels by preventing frequent spikes and crashes. Stable blood sugar levels contribute to better energy management and reduced cravings for sugary or high-calorie foods.

8. **<u>Promotion of Healthy Eating Patterns</u>**: The structure of a 17-hour fasting window encourages mindful eating during the feeding period. This can lead to healthier food choices and portion control, supporting weight loss goals.

9. **<u>Balanced Hormones</u>**: Fasting can contribute to the balance of hormones involved in weight regulation, such as leptin. Balanced hormonal activity supports a more controlled appetite and energy balance.

10. **<u>Preservation of Lean Muscle Mass</u>**: Unlike prolonged fasting, a 17-hour fasting window is generally short enough to preserve lean muscle mass. This is important for maintaining overall metabolic health during weight loss.

11. **Long-Term Sustainability**: The 17-hour fasting approach is considered more sustainable for many individuals compared to more restrictive diets. It allows for flexibility in food choices while still promoting weight loss over the long term.

It's essential to note that individual responses to fasting can vary, and consulting with a healthcare professional before making significant changes to one's eating patterns is advisable, especially for those with pre-existing health conditions.

Understanding the Autophagy Process in Humans

17-Hour Water Fasting Book Guide for Weight Loss, Anti-Aging, Detoxing, and Inner Cells Healing

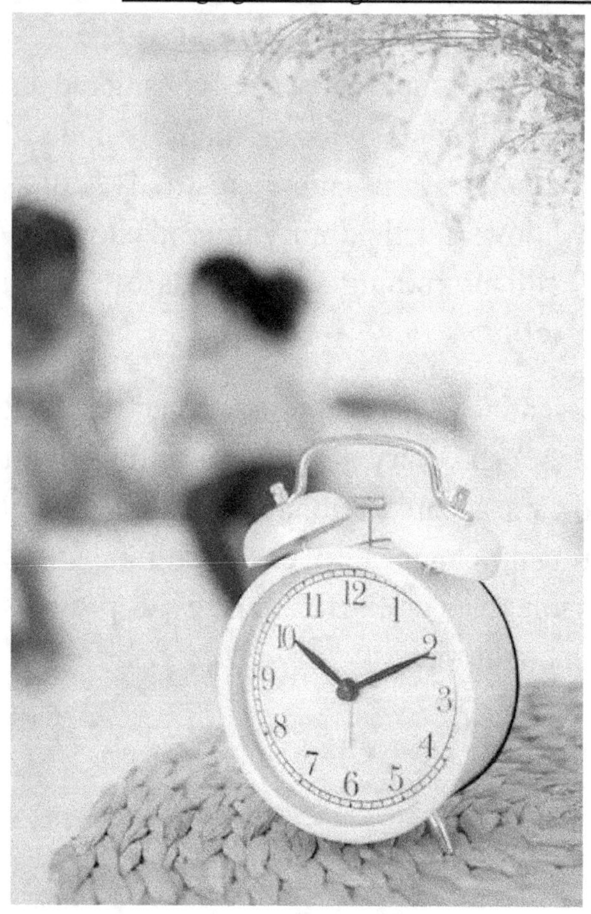

Chapter 2: Anti-Aging Strategies Through Autophagy

The most compelling aspect of anti-aging strategies through autophagy lies in the profound impact this cellular process has on promoting longevity, vitality, and the overall slowing down of the aging process.

Let's explore the key elements that make autophagy a fascinating and effective approach to counteract aging:

→ **Cellular Renewal and Rejuvenation**: Autophagy serves as a natural fountain of youth for cells. By selectively removing damaged cellular components and recycling them, autophagy facilitates cellular renewal and rejuvenation. This continual self-cleansing process contributes to maintaining cellular health over time.

→ **Mitigation of Cellular Stress**: Aging is associated with an accumulation of cellular stress and damage. Autophagy acts as a powerful stress response mechanism, efficiently clearing away misfolded proteins, dysfunctional organelles, and other stress-inducing elements. This mitigation of cellular stress is instrumental in promoting a more resilient cellular environment.

→ **DNA Repair and Genomic Stability**: Autophagy plays a role in DNA repair processes, contributing to the preservation of genomic stability. As DNA damage is a hallmark of aging, the ability of autophagy to aid in repairing genetic material is a crucial aspect of its anti-aging effects.

→ **Prevention of Cellular Senescence**: Cellular senescence, where cells lose their ability to divide and function properly, is a hallmark of aging. Autophagy has been linked to the prevention of cellular senescence, maintaining a balance that supports the longevity and functionality of cells.

→ **Enhanced Mitochondrial Function via Mitophagy**: Autophagy's role in mitophagy, the selective removal of damaged mitochondria, is pivotal for maintaining energy production and cellular function. By promoting healthy mitochondrial function, autophagy contributes to sustained vitality and resilience against aging-related energy decline.

→ **Regulation of Inflammation**: Chronic inflammation is closely associated with aging and age-related diseases. Autophagy helps regulate inflammation by removing inflamed cellular components. This anti-inflammatory effect contributes to a healthier aging process.

→ **Optimized Cellular Metabolism**: Autophagy influences cellular metabolism, promoting a balance between energy production and consumption. This optimization of metabolic processes is crucial for preventing metabolic disorders and promoting overall well-being as the body ages.

→ **Neuroprotective Effects**: Autophagy is particularly significant in the brain, where it plays a role in clearing protein aggregates associated with neurodegenerative diseases. The neuroprotective effects of autophagy contribute to maintaining cognitive function and preventing age-related decline in brain health.

→ **Longevity and Extended Healthspan**: Perhaps the most captivating aspect is the potential for autophagy to contribute to increased longevity and an extended health span. By supporting cellular health and resilience, autophagy may help individuals age more gracefully, enjoying a higher quality of life in their later years.

In summary, the best part of anti-aging strategies through autophagy lies in their holistic and multifaceted approach to maintaining cellular health. From DNA repair to stress mitigation and enhanced energy production, autophagy emerges as a powerful ally in the quest for graceful aging and an extended period of vibrant well-being.

Practical Breakdown of Autophagy Process and 17-Hour Water Fasting for Health Benefits:

Autophagy Process

→ <u>**Initiation**</u>:

1. **How**: *Nutrient scarcity, triggered by fasting or caloric restriction, inhibits mTOR, initiating autophagy.*
2. **Benefits**: *Selective removal of damaged cellular components.*

→ <u>**Autophagosome Formation**</u>:

1. **How**: *Autophagosomes engulf cellular material slated for degradation.*
2. **Benefits**: *Cellular cleansing and recycling.*

→ <u>**Lysosomal Degradation**</u>:

1. **How**: *Autophagosomes fuse with lysosomes, where degradation occurs.*

2. **Benefits**: *Breakdown of cellular debris into basic building blocks.*

➔ <u>**Mitophagy**</u>:
1. **How**: *Selective removal of damaged mitochondria.*
2. **Benefits**: *Improved mitochondrial health and energy production.*

➔ <u>**DNA Repair and Genomic Stability**</u>:
1. **How**: *Autophagy contributes to the repair of damaged DNA.*
2. **Benefits**: *Preservation of genomic integrity.*

➔ **Reduction in Inflammation**:
1. **How**: *Autophagy removes inflamed cellular components.*
2. **Benefits**: *Anti-inflammatory effects, supporting overall health.*

17-Hour Water Fasting for Health Benefits

→ <u>**Weight Loss**</u>:

1. **How**: *Fasting induces fat burning as glycogen stores are depleted.*
2. **Benefits**: *Efficient weight loss without the need for strict dieting.*

→ <u>**Anti-Aging**</u>:

1. **How**: *Fasting activates autophagy, supporting mitochondrial health, DNA repair, and inflammation reduction.*
2. **Benefits**: *It slows down the aging process, promoting longevity.*

→ <u>**Detoxing**</u>:

1. **How**: *Fasting reduces oxidative stress, activates detoxification pathways in the liver, and supports autophagy-driven cellular cleansing.*
2. **Benefits**: *Systemic detoxification at cellular and organ levels.*

➔ **<u>Inner Cells Healing</u>:**

1. **How**: *Autophagy promotes the removal of damaged cellular components, contributing to cellular renewal and regeneration.*

2. **Benefits**: *Healing at the cellular level, enhancing overall well-being.*

Foods and Fruits Before and After Fasting

→ Before Fasting:

1. **Low-Glycemic Foods**: *Opt for foods with a low glycemic index to avoid rapid blood sugar spikes. Examples include leafy greens, non-starchy vegetables, and legumes.*

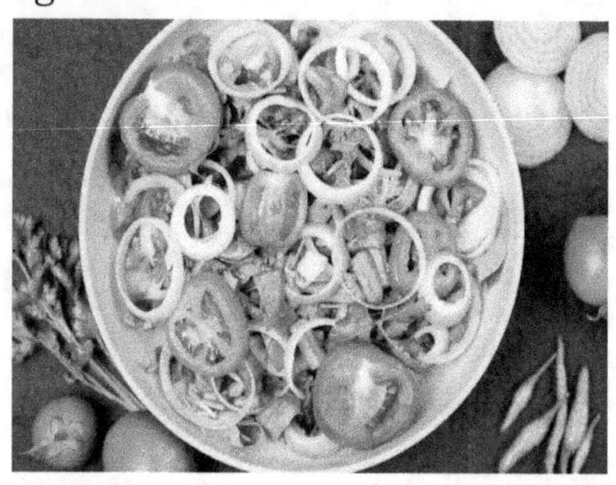

Understanding the Autophagy Process in Humans

17-Hour Water Fasting Book Guide for Weight Loss, Anti-Aging, Detoxing, and Inner Cells Healing

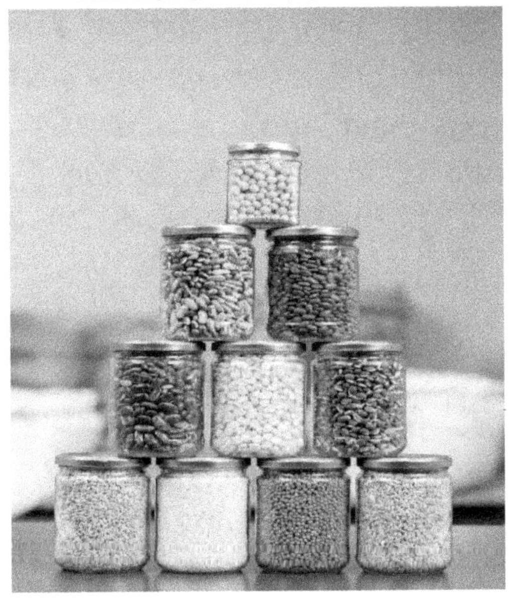

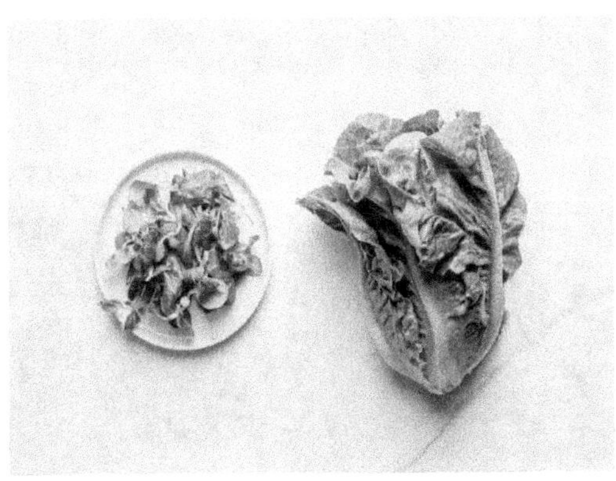

2. **Healthy Fats**: *Incorporate sources of healthy fats, such as avocados, nuts, seeds, and olive oil. These provide sustained energy during fasting.*

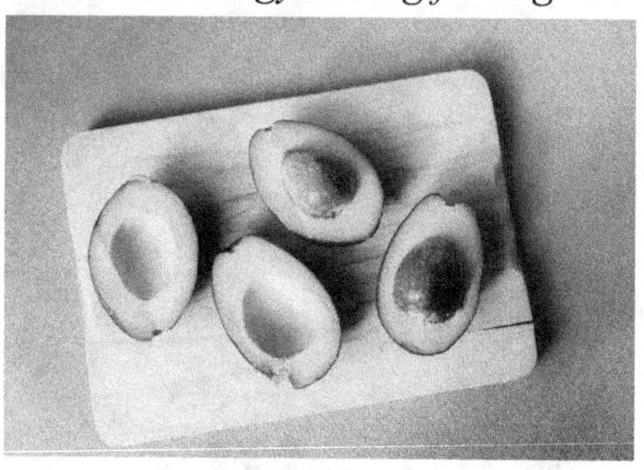

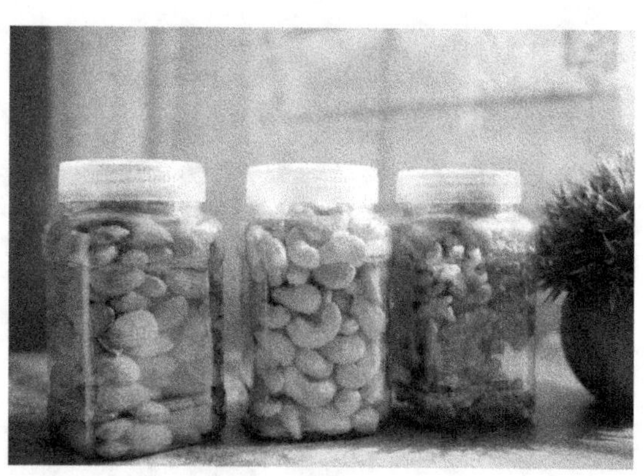

Understanding the Autophagy Process in Humans
17-Hour Water Fasting Book Guide for Weight Loss, Anti-Aging, Detoxing, and Inner Cells Healing

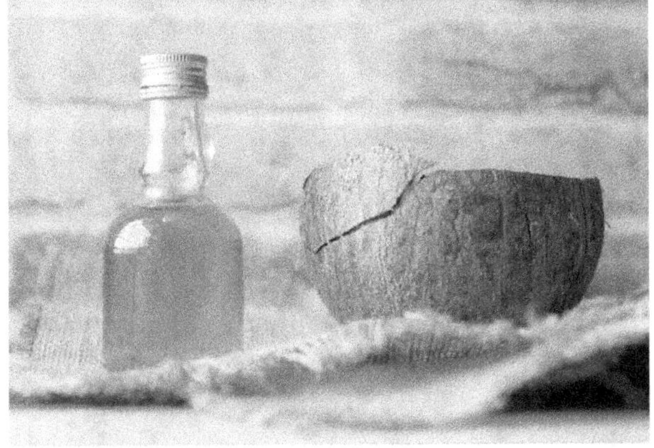

3. **Protein-rich foods**: *Consume lean proteins like poultry, fish, tofu, or legumes to support muscle maintenance during fasting.*

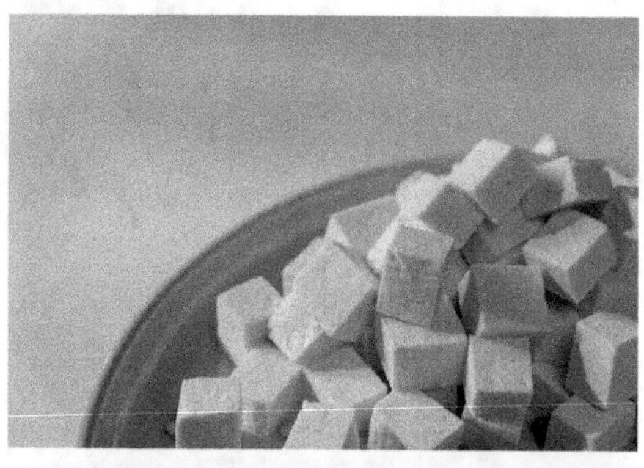

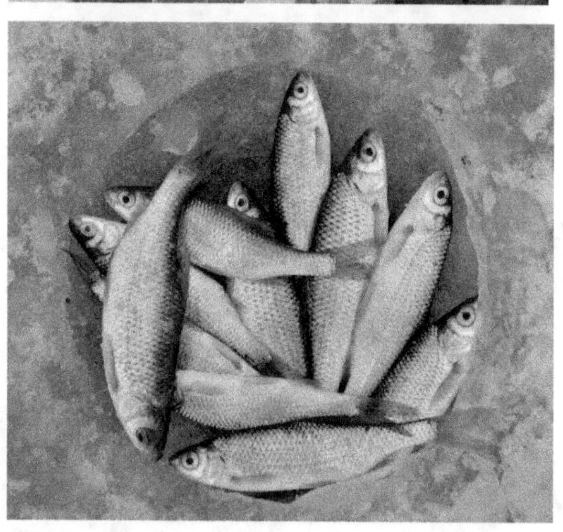

4. Hydrating Foods: *Include foods with high water content, such as cucumbers, watermelon, and celery, to stay hydrated.*

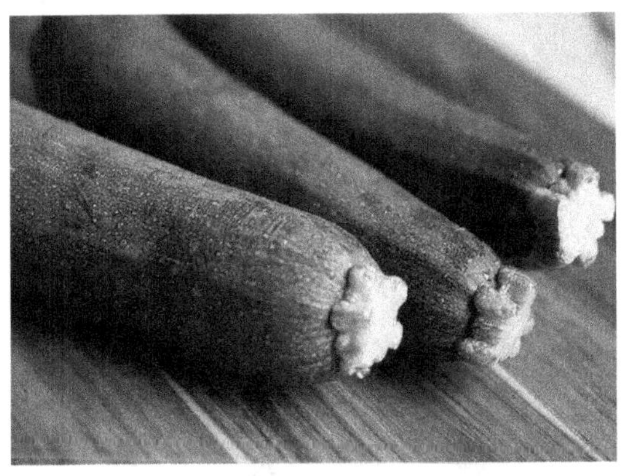

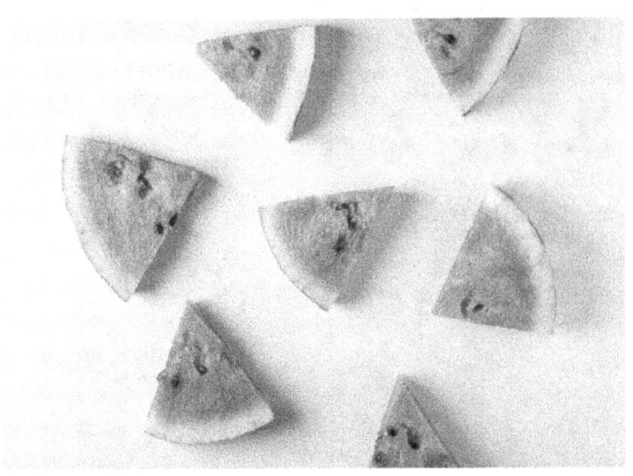

After Fasting

1. **Bone Broth**: *A nutrient-rich option containing amino acids and minerals to support recovery.*

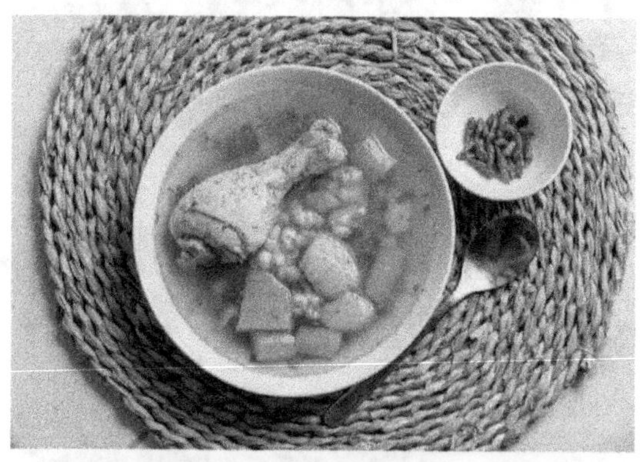

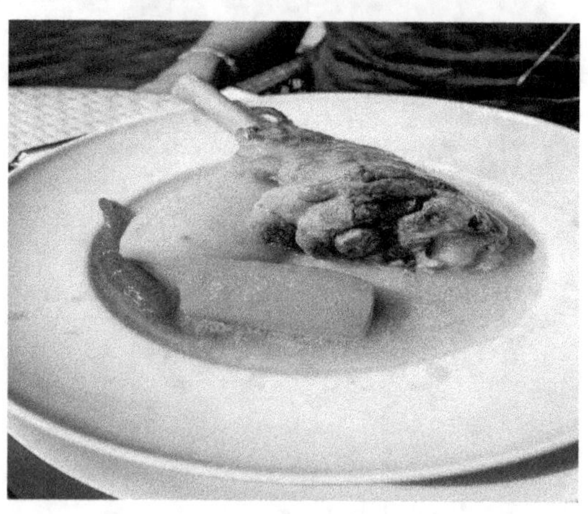

2. **Protein-Rich Meals**: *Include lean proteins to replenish amino acids and support muscle repair.*

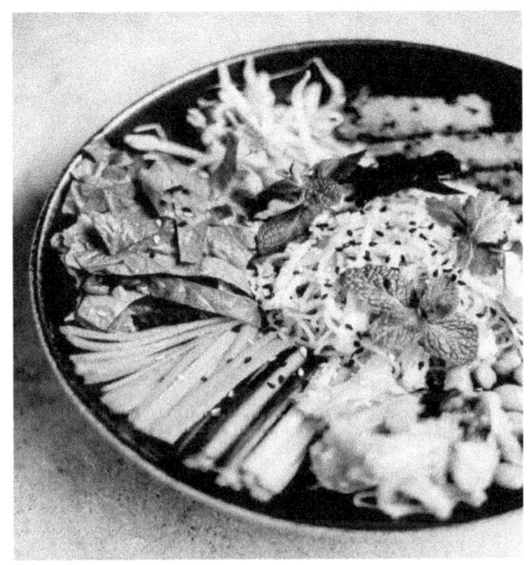

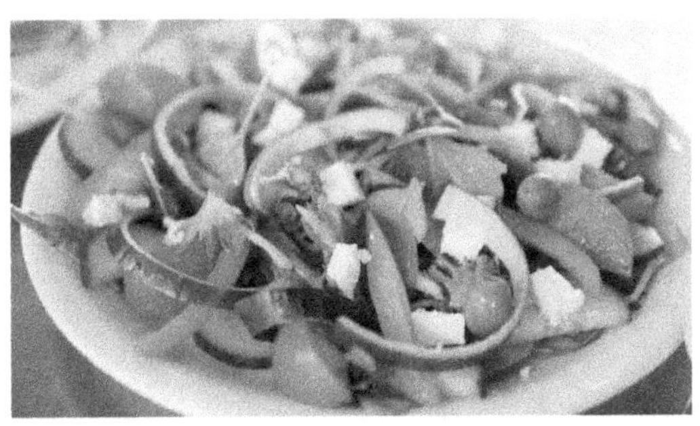

3. Leafy Greens and Vegetables: *Rich in vitamins and minerals, promoting overall health.*

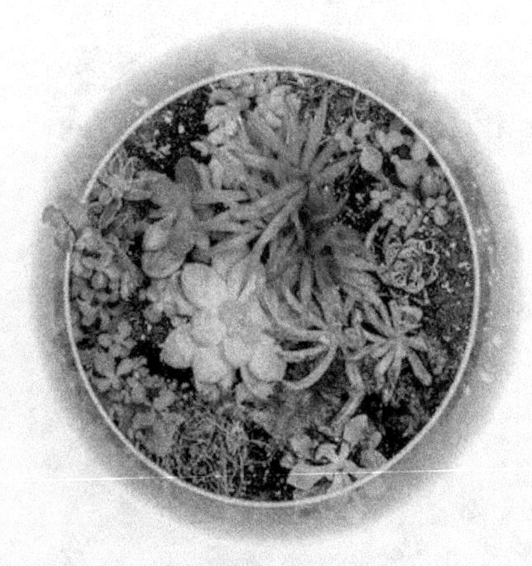

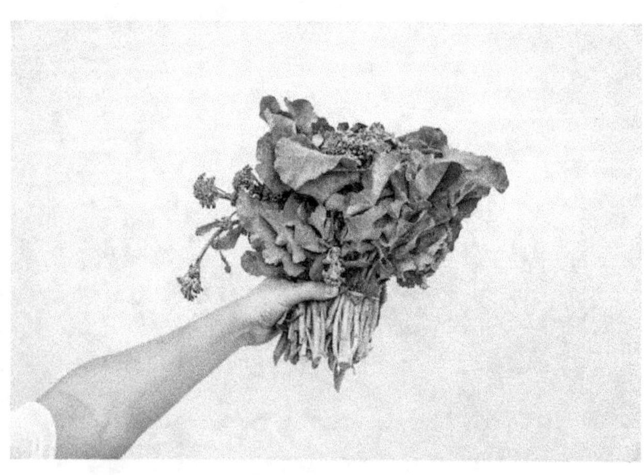

4. Berries: *Berries are low in sugar and high in antioxidants, providing a healthy dessert option.*

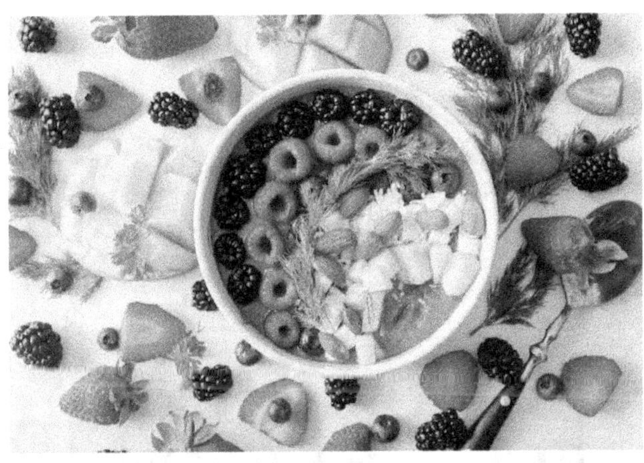

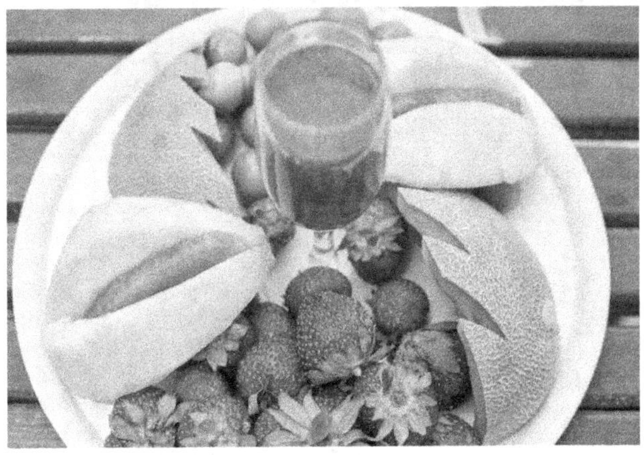

5. **Probiotic Foods**: *Support gut health with yogurt, kefir, or fermented foods.*

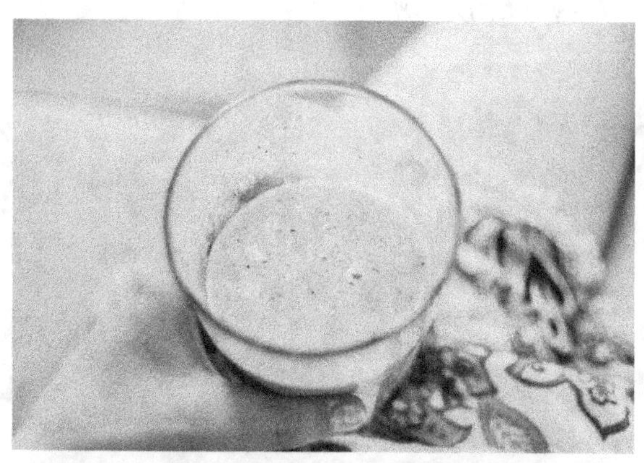

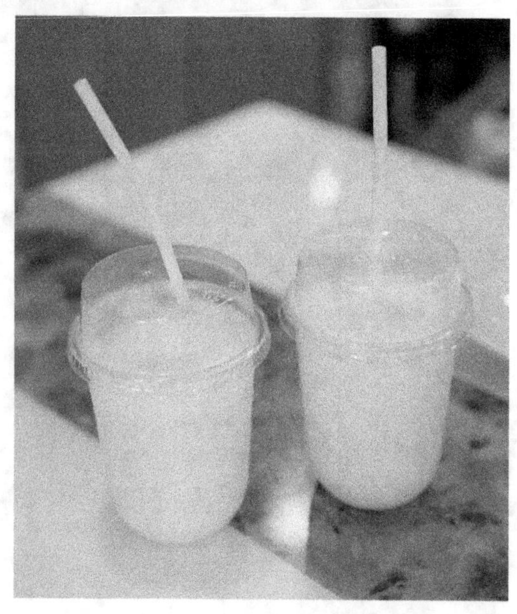

Remember to break your fast gently, gradually reintroducing regular meals to avoid digestive discomfort. It's essential to listen to your body and make food choices that align with your health goals. Consulting a healthcare professional before making significant changes to your diet is advisable, especially for those with pre-existing health conditions.

Testimonials and Case Studies on Anti-Aging Benefits

Increased Energy and Vitality:

→ **Testimonial**: "After adopting intermittent fasting into my daily activities, I saw a substantial increase in vitality and mental clarity. I feel more rejuvenated and ready to take on the day, which has positively impacted both my personal and professional life."

Youthful Skin and Improved Complexion:

→ **Case Study**: "In an intermittent fasting study, patients reported greater skin health, mainly a more youthful skin appearance." The fasting period seemed to stimulate collagen production, leading to visibly smoother and healthier skin."

Weight Loss and Body Composition Improvements:

→ **Testimonial**: "I struggled with weight management for years, but since adopting a 17-hour fasting window, I've experienced significant weight loss and improvements in body composition. It's not just about the numbers on the scale; my overall physique feels more toned and resilient."

Cognitive Sharpness and Mental Clarity:

→ **Case Study**: "A study examining the cognitive benefits of fasting revealed enhanced mental clarity and improved cognitive function in participants. Fasting appeared to support neuroplasticity and protect against age-related cognitive decline."

Reduced Joint Pain and Inflammation:

→ **Testimonial**: "I experienced significant joint soreness for years, but shortly after intermittent fasting, the inflammation subsided dramatically. The anti-inflammatory effects of fasting have made a noticeable difference in my overall comfort and joint health."

Balanced Blood Sugar Levels:

→ **Case Study**: "Those who took part with prediabetes and underwent intermittent fasting observed improvements in insulin sensitivity and balanced blood sugar levels." This not only reduces the risk of diabetes but also contributes to overall anti-aging benefits."

Enhanced Longevity Markers:

➔ **Testimonial**: "As someone in my 50s, I was looking for ways to support longevity and healthy aging. Intermittent fasting has become a cornerstone of my lifestyle, and the improvements in my biomarkers, such as cholesterol levels and blood pressure, are indicative of its anti-aging effects."

Improved Sleep Quality:

➔ **Case Study**: "In a study exploring the effects of intermittent fasting on sleep, participants reported improved sleep quality and patterns. Better sleep is a crucial factor in promoting overall health and supporting the body's natural anti-aging processes."

Stress Reduction and Emotional Well-being:

➔ **Testimonial**: "Fasting has not only positively impacted my physical health but has also been a game-changer for stress reduction and emotional well-being.

I feel more resilient and more prepared to deal with life's obstacles."

Muscle Tone Preservation:

→ **Case Study**: "People who included intermittent fasting into their training routines maintained muscular tone while losing weight. This suggests that fasting may promote fat loss while minimizing muscle loss, contributing to a more youthful physique."

Heart Health Improvement:

→ **Testimonial**: "My journey with intermittent fasting has led to noticeable improvements in heart health markers. My cholesterol levels have normalized, and I feel confident that I am taking proactive steps towards cardiovascular well-being."

These testimonials and case studies provide compelling insights into the diverse anti-aging benefits reported by individuals practicing intermittent fasting. While individual responses may vary, these real-life experiences and scientific investigations highlight the potential positive impact of fasting on various aspects of health and aging.

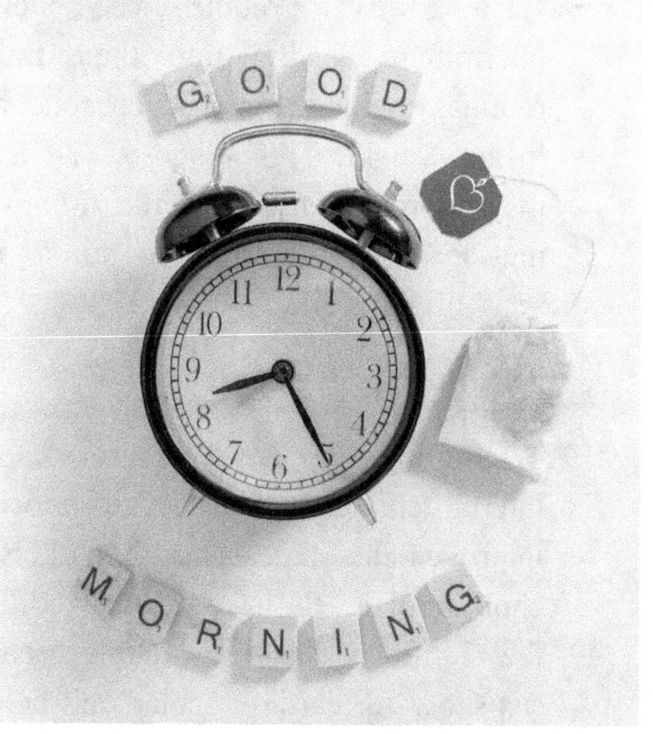

Chapter 3: Detoxing and Inner Cells Healing with Extended Fasting

Extended fasting, such as the practice of 17-hour water fast, can initiate a profound detoxification and inner cell healing process within the human body. This process involves a series of intricate mechanisms that contribute to cleansing at both the cellular and systemic levels.

Let's delve into the journey of detoxing and inner cell healing during extended fasting:

→ **Autophagy Initiation**: The cornerstone of detoxification and inner cell healing is the activation of autophagy. Extended fasting, characterized by a significant reduction in nutrient intake, triggers the upregulation of autophagy. This cellular process involves the targeted removal and recycling of damaged or dysfunctional cellular components, contributing to inner cell cleansing.

→ **Cellular Cleansing and Recycling**: Autophagy facilitates the formation of autophagosomes, specialized vesicles that encapsulate cellular material slated for degradation. These autophagosomes then fuse with lysosomes, where the cellular components are broken down into basic building blocks. This recycling process not only detoxifies the cell but also provides raw materials for the synthesis of new and healthy cellular structures.

→ **Mitophagy for Mitochondrial Health**: A crucial aspect of inner cell healing involves mitophagy, a specific form of autophagy targeting mitochondria. Mitochondria are the energy producers of the cell, and during extended fasting, damaged mitochondria are selectively removed. This enhances energy production and reduces oxidative stress, contributing to inner cell healing.

→ **Reduction in Oxidative Stress**: Fasting leads to a reduction in oxidative stress, a state where the balance between free radicals and antioxidants is disturbed. By limiting the intake of external sources of oxidative stress (such as certain foods), and promoting the removal of damaged cellular components through autophagy, fasting contributes to a detoxifying effect and mitigates oxidative damage.

→ **Elimination of Cellular Waste Products**: Extended fasting stimulates the elimination of accumulated cellular waste products. As autophagy engages in the breakdown of cellular debris, the resulting by-products are efficiently removed from the cell. This detoxifying process helps maintain a cleaner cellular environment.

→ **Enhanced Detoxification Pathways**: Fasting supports the activation of detoxification pathways in the liver. The liver plays a central role in processing and eliminating toxins from the body. During fasting, the liver is given an opportunity to focus on detoxification, aiding in the removal of accumulated toxins from the bloodstream.

→ **Cellular Renewal and Regeneration**: Beyond detoxification, extended fasting promotes cellular renewal and regeneration. As damaged components are cleared away, the cell undergoes a rejuvenation process. This contributes to overall inner cell healing and supports the maintenance of healthy and functional cells.

→ **Hormetic Response and Cellular Resilience**: Extended fasting induces a hormetic response, where cells experience a beneficial stressor that prompts an adaptive response. This stressor, in the form of fasting, enhances cellular resilience. Cells become better equipped to withstand future stressors, promoting long-term inner cell health.

→ **Anti-Inflammatory Effects**: Fasting is associated with a reduction in inflammatory markers. Chronic inflammation is a contributor to various health issues, and by lowering inflammation, extended fasting supports a less inflammatory and more healing cellular environment.

→ **Balancing Hormones for Cellular Harmony**: Fasting influences hormone levels, promoting a state of balance. Hormones related to metabolism, stress response, and cellular regulation are optimized during fasting, contributing to a harmonious and healing cellular environment.

In summary, the process of detoxing and inner cell healing during extended fasting involves the orchestration of various cellular mechanisms. Autophagy, mitophagy, reduction in oxidative stress, and enhanced detoxification pathways collectively contribute to a comprehensive cleansing and renewal process, promoting inner cell health and vitality.

Understanding Detoxification Processes in the Body

Detoxification refers to the process of removing toxins from the body. These toxins can come from various sources, such as food, environmental pollutants, medications, or alcohol. Understanding detoxification processes in the body is essential for maintaining optimal health and preventing various diseases.

The Role of the Liver:

The liver plays a crucial role in detoxification. It is the main organ responsible for breaking down toxins, converting them into less harmful compounds, and then eliminating them from the body. The liver has four stages of detoxification, which include:

1. **Phase 1**: In this stage, toxins are converted into more reactive compounds

with the help of enzymes. This prepares them for the following step.

2. **Phase 2**: During this stage, additional enzymes further modify and detoxify the toxins. This helps to make them more water-soluble and easier to excrete.

3. **Phase 3**: In this final stage, the toxins are transported out of the liver via bile or urine, depending on the specific compound.

The Importance of Detoxification:

Detoxification is essential for the body to function optimally. It helps to protect the liver and kidneys from damage, improves overall liver function, and enhances immune function. By removing toxins from the body, detoxification also helps prevent chronic diseases such as liver disease, kidney disease, and certain types of cancer.

Factors Affecting Detoxification

Several factors can influence the effectiveness of detoxification in the body. These include:

- **Eating Habits**: A diet high in processed foods, sugar, and unhealthy fats can hinder detoxification processes. A nutritious and balanced diet rich in fruits, vegetables, whole grains, and lean proteins can support detoxification.

- **Excessive Alcohol Consumption**: Excessive alcohol consumption can damage the liver and reduce the body's ability to detoxify. It is important to moderate alcohol intake or avoid it altogether.

- **Vitamins and Minerals**: Certain vitamins and minerals, such as vitamin C, vitamin E, selenium, and zinc, are essential for efficient detoxification. Getting enough of these nutrients through food sources or supplements can help support the body's detoxification processes.

- **Exercise**: Regular exercise helps increase blood flow and improve circulation, which facilitates the distribution and elimination of toxins. Engaging in activities such as walking, yoga, or strength training can be beneficial for detoxification.

- **Rest and Relaxation**: Adequate rest and stress management are vital for effective detoxification. Chronic stress can impair liver function and disrupt detoxification pathways. Incorporating relaxation techniques such as yoga, meditation, or deep breathing can help promote detoxification.

Understanding detoxification processes in the body is crucial for maintaining optimal health. The liver plays a central role in this process, breaking down toxins and converting them into less harmful substances. Factors such as diet, alcohol consumption, exercise, and stress management all influence the body's ability to detoxify effectively. By paying attention to these factors and adopting a healthy lifestyle, individuals can help promote detoxification and support the body's natural cleansing processes.

Practical Tips and Guidance for Safe Extended Fasting

Practical Tips and Guidance for Safe Extended Fasting refers to a set of guidelines and best practices aimed at ensuring the safety of individuals who engage in extended fasting, also known as prolonged fasting.

Prolonged fasting refers to the practice of voluntarily abstaining from food for an extended period, typically lasting between 24 and 48 hours. While extended fasting has gained attention in recent years for its potential benefits, it is crucial to follow safety precautions to prevent any potential health risks.

When engaging in extended fasting, our bodies undergo various metabolic changes, which can impact various physiological functions. Our bodies rely on a steady supply of nutrients from food to maintain optimal function, and prolonged fasting disrupts this balance. By following practical tips and guidance, individuals can minimize the risks and maximize the potential benefits of extended fasting.

One of the key considerations during extended fasting is hydration. Drinking an adequate amount of water is crucial to prevent dehydration, which can have detrimental effects on the body. It is recommended to stay hydrated by consuming an adequate amount of water throughout the day, even during the fasting period. Water also helps to regulate body temperature and flush out toxins.

Another aspect of practical guidance for safe extended fasting is maintaining a balanced diet before and after the fasting period. While fasting, it is important to focus on consuming nutrient-rich foods that promote overall health and well-being. This entails consuming plenty of fruits and vegetables, entire grains, lean meats, and healthy fats. Prioritizing nutrition before and after fasting can help support the body's basic functions and recovery during the fasting period.

Additionally, it is advisable to incorporate regular physical activity into your daily routine, even during fasting. Moderate-intensity exercise, such as walking or light jogging, can help improve insulin sensitivity, regulate blood sugar levels, and promote overall well-being. However, it is crucial to avoid engaging in intense exercise or excessive physical activity during prolonged fasting, as it can lead to imbalances in energy stores and potential health risks.

Furthermore, it is important to listen to your body and adjust your fasting practices accordingly. Each person's response to extended fasting is unique, and it is essential to be aware of any physical discomfort or potential risks.

Consulting with a medical professional or a registered dietitian can provide personalized advice tailored to your specific needs.

In conclusion, "Practical Tips and Guidance for Safe Extended Fasting" refers to a set of guidelines and best practices aimed at ensuring the safety of individuals who engage in prolonged fasting. By following these practical tips, individuals can minimize the risks associated with extended fasting and maximize its potential health benefits. It is essential to stay hydrated, maintain a balanced diet, incorporate regular physical activity, and pay attention to your body's response to fasting.

Chapter 4: Smoothies to Support the 17-Hour Water-Fasting

Creating autophagy-supporting smoothies for a 17-hour water-fasting period involves selecting nutrient-dense ingredients that nourish the body while keeping calorie intake minimal.

Here are five different smoothie ideas designed to complement the autophagy process during fasting:

Green Detox Smoothie

- ❖ **Ingredients:**
  - → **Spinach or kale**: *Rich in chlorophyll and antioxidants.*
  - → **Cucumber**: *Hydrating and low in calories.*
  - → **Celery**: *Provides electrolytes and supports hydration.*
  - → **Lemon juice**: *Adds a refreshing flavor and vitamin C.*

→ **Ginger**: *Anti-inflammatory properties.*

❖ **Explanation:**

→ This smoothie is packed with green, leafy vegetables that are low in calories but high in essential nutrients. The combination of hydrating ingredients and antioxidants supports the detoxification process and provides a refreshing drink during fasting.

Berry Antioxidant Blend

❖ **Ingredients:**
→ **Mixed berries (blueberries, raspberries, strawberries)**: *Rich in antioxidants.*
→ **Chia seeds**: *Provide fiber and omega-3 fatty acids.*
→ **Almond milk**: *Adds a creamy texture without containing excess calories.*
→ **Flaxseeds**: *Source of fiber and anti-inflammatory omega-3s.*
→ **Cinnamon**: *Adds flavor and may have anti-inflammatory effects.*

❖ **Explanation:**

→ Berries are antioxidant powerhouses that can enhance autophagy. The chia seeds and flaxseeds provide additional fiber for satiety, and the almond milk contributes creaminess without adding many calories.

Avocado Protein Smoothie

❖ **Ingredients:**

→ **Avocado**: *Healthy fats for sustained energy.*

→ **Spinach**: *Rich in chlorophyll and nutrients.*

→ **Protein powder (plant-based)**: *Supports muscle maintenance.*

→ **Unsweetened coconut water**: *Provides electrolytes.*

→ **Mint leaves**: *Adds a refreshing flavor.*

❖ **Explanation:**

→ Avocado provides healthy fats and a creamy texture, while the protein powder supports muscle maintenance during fasting. The coconut water contributes electrolytes for hydration, and the mint adds a refreshing touch.

Turmeric Spice Elixir

* **Ingredients:**
- **Turmeric (fresh or powdered)**: *Anti-inflammatory properties.*
- **Ginger**: *Adds a zesty kick and has anti-inflammatory benefits.*
- **Coconut milk**: *Provides healthy fats and a rich flavor.*
- **Black pepper**: *Enhances the absorption of turmeric.*
- **Stevia or monk fruit (optional)**: *For a touch of sweetness without calories.*

* **Explanation:**

- This anti-inflammatory elixir incorporates turmeric and ginger, known for their health-promoting properties. The addition of black pepper enhances the bioavailability of turmeric, and coconut milk provides a creamy base.

Citrus Immunity Booster

- ❖ **Ingredients:**
- → **Oranges or grapefruits**: *High in vitamin C and antioxidants.*
- → **Carrots**: *Rich in beta-carotene and vitamins.*
- → **Lemon juice**: *Adds a citrusy flavor and vitamin C.*
- → **Greek yogurt (optional)**: *Adds protein and creaminess.*
- → **Ice cubes**: *For a refreshing texture.*

- ❖ **Explanation:**

- → Citrus fruits are rich in vitamin C and antioxidants, supporting the immune system. Carrots add additional vitamins and beta-carotene. Greek yogurt can be included for added protein and a creamier consistency.

Tips for Autophagy-Supporting Smoothies:

→ **Keep it low-Calorie**: Aim for nutrient-dense ingredients with minimal calories to support autophagy without breaking the fast.

→ **Stay Hydrated**: Incorporate hydrating ingredients like cucumber, coconut water, or ice cubes to support hydration during fasting.

→ **Include Antioxidants**: Berries, leafy greens, and citrus fruits are rich in antioxidants that may enhance autophagy.

→ **Experiment with Herbs and Spices**: Ingredients like ginger, turmeric, mint, and cinnamon not only add flavor but also contribute to anti-inflammatory benefits.

Remember to listen to your body and adjust ingredients based on personal preferences and sensitivities. Consulting with a healthcare professional before introducing new ingredients into your diet, especially during fasting, is advisable, especially for those with pre-existing health conditions.

Conclusion

In concluding the exploration of the book "*Understanding the Autophagy Process in Humans: 17-Hour Water Fasting Book Guide for Weight Loss, Anti-Aging, Detoxing, and Inner Cells Healing*," it becomes evident that the autophagy process is a remarkable and multifaceted tool for enhancing overall health and well-being. The book has unveiled the intricacies of autophagy, illustrating its pivotal role in weight loss, anti-aging, detoxification, and the profound healing of inner cells.

Summary of Key Takeaways:

- *Autophagy as a Cellular Rejuvenation Mechanism*: Autophagy emerges as a powerful cellular rejuvenation mechanism, facilitating the removal of damaged components and promoting cellular renewal.

- ***17-Hour Water Fasting for Weight Loss***: The book emphasizes the benefits of a 17-hour water fasting regimen, showcasing its effectiveness in weight loss through mechanisms like enhanced fat burning and improved metabolic health.

- ***Anti-Aging Strategies Through Autophagy:*** Autophagy proves to be a key player in anti-aging strategies, contributing to mitochondrial health, DNA repair, inflammation reduction, and the overall promotion of longevity.

- ***Detoxing and Inner Cells Healing:*** Extended fasting, as highlighted in the book, initiates a detoxification process at both the cellular and systemic levels. Autophagy-driven inner cell healing involves the removal of cellular waste and the optimization of detoxification pathways.

Encouragement for Implementing Autophagy for Health:

As readers conclude their journey through this insightful guide, the encouragement to implement autophagy for health is paramount. The book serves as a roadmap, offering practical insights into how a 17-hour water fasting approach can be seamlessly integrated into one's lifestyle. It empowers individuals to take charge of their health by leveraging the natural and potent benefits of autophagy.

The encouragement lies in the recognition that autophagy is not a complex or elusive process but a natural mechanism that can be harnessed through mindful fasting. Implementing the principles outlined in the book holds the promise of weight management, anti-aging effects, detoxification, and a profound healing of inner cells.

In adopting these practices, individuals embark on a journey towards a healthier and more resilient life. The book stands as a guide, urging readers to embrace the transformative power of autophagy, fostering a renewed sense of vitality and well-being. It is an invitation to not only understand the science behind autophagy but to actively incorporate its principles, unlocking the potential for a healthier, rejuvenated, and more fulfilling life.

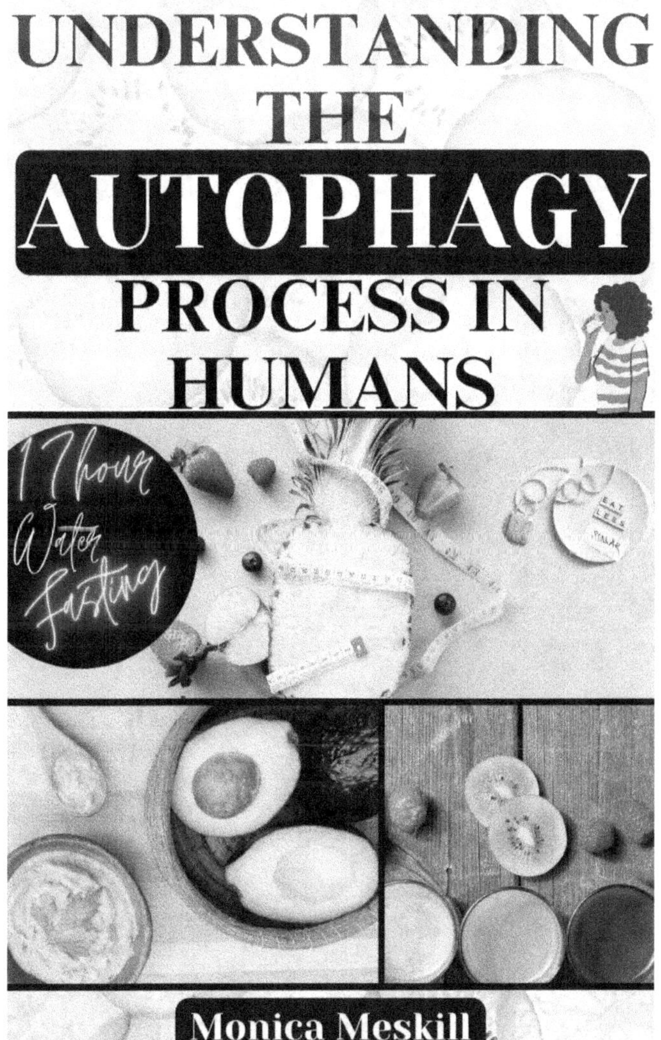
UNDERSTANDING
THE
AUTOPHAGY
PROCESS IN
HUMANS
17 hour
Water
Fasting
Monica Meskill

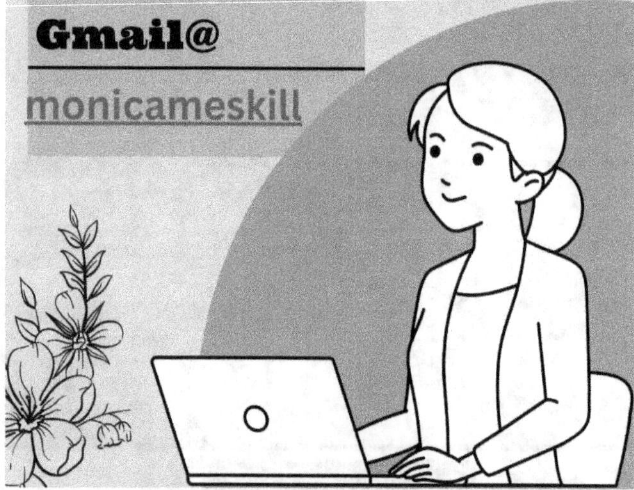
WHAT SHOULD WE IMPROVE?
GIVE US
YOUR FEEDBACK
REALLY IMPORTANT
Gmail@
monicameskill
monicameskill@gmail.com

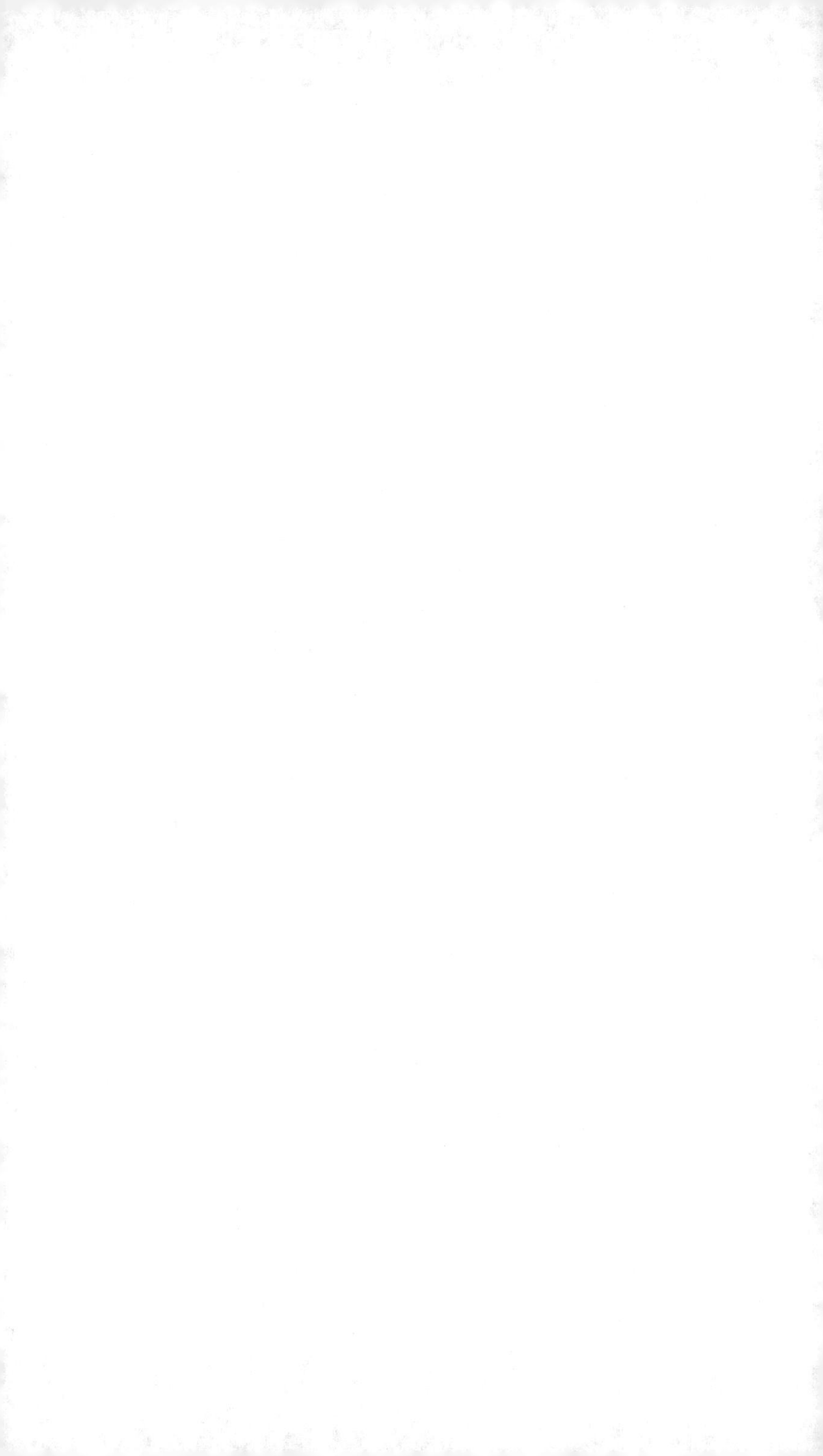